Stephanie Berryman

Nine Strategies for Dealing with Workplace Stress

D1508811

Practical Tools
to Reduce and Manage
Workplace Stress

Contents

Dedication:

This book is dedicated to the close friends I have made at work – Lauri Thompson and Gerhard Maynard – you are friends who have become family, Godparents to my children and a godsend to Andrew and I. Your friendship has made both my work and my life richer.

Invitation:

Thank you so much for buying my book. I hope it provides you with practical strategies to help you reduce your work-related stress. If you are interested in hearing more about my experiences and perspective, please join me at Stephanieberryman.com or follow me on Medium https://medium.com/@stephanieberry. I write about how we can live good lives, no matter what our circumstances are. Get my free e-book 'The Good Life Manifesto'. If you'd like to learn more about my leadership consulting and coaching, please visit my website – www.managetoengage.com.

Other Books in This Series:
9 Strategies for Dealing with Stress
9 Strategies for Dealing with the Difficult Stuff

Nine Strategies for Dealing with Workplace Stress

Welcome to my little book of strategies to help you manage and reduce your workplace stress. It's short because I know you don't have much time – and I like to write practical books that get right to the point. Every strategy in this book has been tried and tested through my work as a leadership development consultant, trainer and coach. I have worked with thousands of people, and I have seen a lot of workplace stress. I also have experienced workplace stress, both as an employee and as a consultant. I've used these strategies myself and taught them to my students and clients and I've seen them work wonders. I'm confident that if you use them, these nine strategies will help you reduce and manage your stress.

Stress is incredibly prevalent in our workplaces today and growing. "85% of Canadian employers and 75% of American employers ranked stress as their top health and productivity concern."[1] A recent report from the National Institute of Occupational Safety and Health found that:

➢ 40% of workers reported their job was very or extremely stressful

➢ 25% view their jobs as the number one stressor in their lives

➢ Three fourths of employees believe that workers have more on-the-job stress than a generation ago

➢ 29% of workers felt quite a bit or extremely stressed at work

➢ Job stress is more strongly associated with health complaints than financial or family problems[2]

Stress is a serious problem. And we are the only ones who can solve it. As much as we would like our workplaces to hire more staff, fire all the difficult people, and give us more time off and better pay, it's not going to happen.

Work will always have some element of stress, and this isn't necessarily a bad thing. We need some level of stress to help us feel motivated and get work done. This is called eustress or "good stress". We don't want to eliminate this energizing stress at work because it keeps us engaged. In contrast, we do want to reduce the negative stress that work generates. Often good stress can shift into negative stress when there is too much of it. It's great to have a project to work

1 https://www.willistowerswatson.com/en-CA/press/2016/06/75-percent-of-us-employers-say-stress-is-top-health-concern
2 https://www.cdc.gov/niosh/docs/99-101/

on and deadlines to work to, but it's not so great to have five projects to work on and five impossible deadlines to meet.

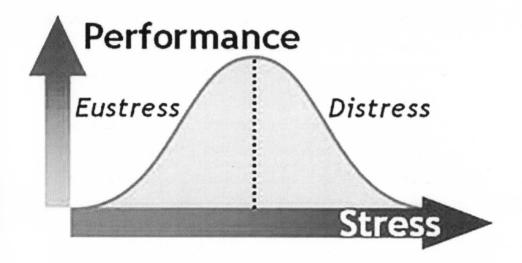

Identify what your stress triggers are as well as what gives you energy. I love autonomy, creative work, helping people, and getting things done. These things make me feel energized and engaged. I dislike and am not very good at paperwork, logistics, or anything to do with technology. I can't avoid those tasks as they are part of my job, but I can minimize how much time I spend on them. I lasted three months in a job as a receptionist because every task that the job required wasn't a strength of mine. I didn't enjoy what I was doing or the environment I was working in – everyone else was stressed out too. I quit, went back to school and found a different job. My new job was a better fit for my natural strengths and was far more satisfying. It can be terrifying to quit but it's worth it to find a job that is right for you. If you have trouble identifying what your strengths and passions are, an excellent and affordable tool to help you do so is the Gallup Strengthsfinder (the link is included in the appendix). It's based on research, accurate and affordable. Knowing your strengths and passions, and working with them, can significantly reduce your negative stress and increase your positive eustress.

We need to pay more attention to our workloads and notice when our "eustress" starts tipping over into stress. Ideally, we want to pull it back as soon as we notice signs that we are feeling stressed out or anxious. The sooner we become aware of this shift, and seek to balance the situation, the easier it is to manage. Most of us know our individual signs of a rising stress level – a kink in the neck, impatience, irritability, difficulty falling asleep, feeling cranky, or frequent headaches. Learn your stress signs, and when you start to see them, do everything you can to reduce your stress.

Unfortunately, many people let their stress pile up and then they end up burned out and exhausted. There are negative consequences of ignoring your stress, including major health issues, relationship breakdown and job loss.

- Working more than 10 hours a day is associated with a 60 percent jump in risk of cardiovascular issues.
- 10 percent of those working 50 to 60 hours report relationship problems; the rate increases to 30 percent for those working more than 60 hours.
- Working more than 40 hours a week is associated with increased alcohol and tobacco consumption, as well as unhealthy weight gain in men and depression in women.
- Little productive work occurs after 50 hours per week[3]

Nothing is worth compromising our health or our relationships. It's crucial that we recognise stress and act to reduce it, as soon as we notice that it is impacting us. Work is only one element of life, and not the most important one. As one of my coaching clients so eloquently put it, you can always find another job but you only have one family.

There are many sources of workplace stress: feeling overwhelmed, feeling disempowered, a lack of clear roles and expectations, an unrealistic workload, workplace politics and interpersonal conflict. It's unlikely that you are going to eliminate all of these sources of negative stress. That is simply reality. Rather than hoping for some fantasy world where there is no stress, what

3 https://www.inc.com/tom-popomaronis/science-says-you-shouldnt-work-more-than-this-number-of-hours-a-day.html

we need are tools to manage these stressors so they don't have as much impact on us.

The strategies I teach are not typical lifestyle tips such as getting more sleep, exercising or meditating. Instead, I focus on the ways we can respond to situations that cause us stress. If you'd like some excellent lifestyle strategies, check out the appendix for additional ideas shared by my readers, colleagues, clients and friends.

While reading this book, I encourage you to choose one or two strategies that might work for you, and start using them right away. I'm confident that you'll see a reduction in your stress. But here's the thing: you actually have to use the strategies. You can't just read them, think they sound good, and then do nothing. This is my first strategy, Take Action, so let's get going.

1. Take action.

We need to start by identifying when a stressor is having a negative impact on our well-being and productivity, and then take action to change things. This book will give you some excellent ideas, but it is your responsibility to take action in order to make changes in your life.

I have coached so many people who feel hopeless about workplace stress. They feel disempowered and frustrated, and continue to allow the stress to impact them. If there is something that causes you stress at work, identify its source and take action. Doing something will reduce your stress even if you don't get the result you were hoping for. You regain your own sense of power when you address stressful situations. Too many people fall into the trap of feeling anxious, and watching the situation get increasingly worse, but doing nothing about it. They put all their focus on their feelings of anxiety and what's stressing them out rather than on what they can do about their challenges. There is always something to be done - we just need to figure out what it is and have the courage to do it.

If you hate your job, start looking for another one. If you don't know how to do a task, ask someone to teach you. If you're underperforming or receiving negative feedback, ask for clear direction on what you need to do to improve and then do it. If you're having difficulty working with someone, have a conversation with them to address and resolve your concerns.

We have control over our circumstances. We can manage many of our stressors by simply addressing them. We have to take action in order to make change. Many of us resist taking action because we fear having difficult conversations. It is worth having an uncomfortable conversation in order to address your concerns and control what you can. The only thing you can control is how you respond to the situation.

Before you race into taking action, stop and carefully assess the situation. Ask yourself the following questions:

Why is this so upsetting for me? This helps you identify what you're feeling and why.

How did I contribute to this? This helps you identify the specific things you did that contributed to the situation.

What can I learn from this? When you focus on learning from the situation, you can focus on growing rather than stressing out.

What can I do about this situation? This helps you focus on specific solutions and strategies.

What can I do differently next time? This helps you identify the specific things you will change in a similar situation in the future.

I once coached a client who was feeling overwhelmed at work; he was certain that his heavy workload was the source of his stress. He started our conversation believing that he needed to decrease his workload and feeling angry that his manager kept piling work on.

As we talked more about the situation, he realised that the way his manager was treating him was actually the source of his stress rather than his workload. His manager continued to give him projects and expected that they would be completed in unrealistic timeframes. In our coaching conversation, he realised that he was contributing to this dynamic by being a "yes" person and taking everything on. It's important to recognise your contribution to the situation because your own behaviour is the easiest thing to change. He needed to recognise and address his own behaviour first, or he would have ended up in the same situation again.

I coached him through having a difficult conversation with his manager. He was nervous but gathered his courage, booked a meeting with her and discussed the situation. He didn't complain that she piled too much work on him. Instead, he started the conversation by taking personal responsibility. He explained that he was taking too much on, and that he kept saying yes instead of no when he was feeling overwhelmed because it was difficult for him to say no. His boss admitted that she had been concerned about the workload but she was relieved that the work was getting done so she just kept asking. Together they prioritized his work, delegated some projects to others, and created a far more manageable workload. In addition to this, their working relationship improved because my client was courageous and vulnerable, and his boss responded in kind.

If my client hadn't taken the time to think through the situation and ask himself what was so upsetting to him and how he had contributed to the situation, he may have taken the wrong approach or addressed the wrong issues. Often when we are stressed out and everything is going at a fast pace, we are too quick to assess the problem and possible solutions. If possible, talk things through with a trusted friend. When you are thinking about the challenge you are dealing with, don't focus on the stress and what's not working.

Take the time to think about the source of your stress, how you are contributing to it, and what action you can take to achieve the best outcome.

Often taking action requires courage. It can be frightening to address a person or situation that is upsetting for you. But it's way better than doing nothing. Many people avoiding dealing with difficult people or situations and hope the problem will magically resolve itself. It won't. Deal with problems as soon as they arise. The longer you wait, the more difficult it becomes.

Whatever your workplace stressor is, be it work overload, lack of clarity, or interpersonal conflicts, you can take initial action by having a conversation and bringing up your concerns. For example, if you don't have clarity about either your role, other people's roles, expectations, direction, priorities or goals, it's okay to ask. Go and ask your direct manager for clarity. Keep asking until you have the information you need. Always do this in a respectful way, approach with curiosity, and recognise that others may be just as stressed out as you are, possibly more.

If your manager can't give you clarity, ask him or her to find out what might be needed so they can get back to you. And if you still can't get clarity, it means the organization and the people above you don't necessarily have clarity either, so go ahead and make things clear for yourself. Set your own goals, priorities and direction.

Years ago, when I went back to work after a maternity leave, I returned to my organization in a new role, one I was excited about. My manager was off on a two-month health leave when I started, and the consultant that was leading my project had to leave unexpectedly. I had no idea what I was expected to do. I was feeling frustrated and uncertain as to how to proceed. I talked to a colleague whose wise advice was, "if they didn't give you direction and there's no one around to clarify things for you, forge your own path." So I did. Taking action reduced my stress and helped me be more productive and engaged. I figured that when my manager returned it was better to show her something rather than admit I had just spun in circles. She was pleased with the work I'd started - we made a few tweaks and I continued working on the project. If you aren't getting the direction you need, set goals that feel relevant to the work, and move towards them. Make sure you keep your manager in the loop, check in frequently, and ask for direction as required.

Whatever the situation that is causing you stress is, take action to resolve it. Even if you don't achieve the outcome you want, taking action empowers you and reduces your stress.

2. Have difficult conversations

One way we can take action is by dealing with difficult interactions that happen at work. Interpersonal conflicts are the most common source of stress I see in workplaces. It can be difficult working with people who have different attitudes, approaches and behaviours than we do. It's possible that you don't feel respected by certain colleagues, or you disagree with their work ethic, maybe you need to work in silence but the person next to you is a chatterbox, or you were sure you were leading the project but a colleague seems determined to take things over.

When dealing with interpersonal conflicts, we need to identify the source of our stress, how we are contributing to it and possible actions we can take. You may not think you are doing anything to contribute to the situation but I promise that you are. Even if it's just by being silent about your frustrations and not addressing the problem, you are contributing to it.

Why is this so upsetting for me? This helps you identify what you're feeling and why.

How did I contribute to this? This helps you identify the specific things you did that contributed to the situation.

What can I learn from this? When you focus on learning from the situation, you can focus on growing rather than stressing out.

What can I do about this situation? This helps you focus on specific solutions and strategies.

What can I do differently next time? This helps you identify the specific things you will change in a similar situation in the future.

An unhealthy workplace behaviour that I see frequently is that when one person has an issue with another person, they don't talk *to* them, they talk *about* them. If you do that, stop. It doesn't resolve the situation, it makes it worse and contributes to a culture of gossip and negativity. If you're really frustrated and need to vent, talk to someone outside of work who can keep the conversation confidential. If it's a situation that has workplace implications and you need to involve your manager, your union rep or HR, do so after you have thought through the situation and you are clear on your part in it, and what kind of support you need.

Many people would rather poke themselves in the eye with a stick than have a difficult conversation. Don't avoid it! I promise you that the sooner you have the conversation, the easier it will be. The longer you leave it, the more frustrated you'll be and the more difficult the situation will be to resolve.

Dealing with interpersonal conflict requires a genuine desire to resolve the situation and find a good outcome for both of you. Now I know, trust me I know, there are some people that are almost impossible to work with. They seem to delight in making life difficult for others. I'm sorry if you have to work with someone like this. If this is the case, the goal is to reduce their impact on you.

There are two ways to do this. You can ignore the behaviour, shrug your shoulders when they engage in difficult behaviour, and think "oh, that's just Bill, doing his thing, nothing to do with me." This is the approach to take if their behaviour is designed to get a reaction from you. When you stop reacting, their behaviour will change. The other response is to address their behaviour. This is the approach to take if you want to let the other person know how they are impacting you with the hope of making changes in how you interact. You will know what action will get you the best result in terms of improving your working relationship.

We can also have conflict and challenges with people that we enjoy working with and we need tools to resolve those challenges. If you decide to have a difficult conversation, I encourage you to use the AIID Feedback model. I've taught this to hundreds of people and I've seen them dramatically change their relationships by using it.

Framework for Feedback - AIID

A	Action – identify the specific action you are giving the person feedback on
I	Impact – share the impact that their action had on you
I	Input – ask for their input
D	Desired outcome – together, come up with a desired outcome to be able to take action on the feedback

First you identify the specific **Action** that is problematic. Here, you have to be as specific as possible – being vague is tempting because you may feel nervous but being specific helps you have a clear conversation.

For example, if someone is not treating you respectfully, you don't want to be vague and say, 'you're being mean to me, or you're not treating me respectfully'. Those are confusing statements and also very likely to make the person feel defensive.

Instead, choose a specific action or behaviour that has occurred in the recent past (1 week). You need to be as specific as possible. You could say, 'in that meeting when you said my idea would never work' or 'when you invited everyone in the office for lunch except me' or 'yesterday, when we were discussing the project roll-out and you interrupted me three times" to provide specific examples to the person you feel is being disrespectful of you.

You need to get very clear on what the behaviour or action is that is difficult for you and be as specific as possible when describing it to the person. Once you are clear on the **Action**, you need to share with the person the **Impact** that their action had on you. This is key. I have seen so many people make significant changes to their behaviour once they became aware of the impact.

In one of my leadership classes, I give students an assignment to go and ask five people for feedback. One of my students had a great insight because people told him that when he was sarcastic, it made them shut down and not want to bring issues to him. He knew that he was sarcastic and prided himself on it, thinking it made him funny and approachable. When he understood the impact of his sarcasm, he changed his behaviour because he wanted to be approachable. We don't know about the impact of our actions unless we ask others or they give us unsolicited feedback. Even though we are hardwired to defend against feedback, if we can get past our initial defense mechanisms, we can learn so much.

Once you've shared the specific Action and the Impact it's had on you, then you ask the other person for their **Input**. There are two questions you can ask at this stage. The first question to ask is "why do you think this is happening?' This helps you both get to the root of the problem and solve it. The next question to ask is "what do you think we can do about it?".

The most important thing to do now is to listen to the other person. Keep in mind that they may be feeling hurt or defensive so it may be difficult for them to engage in the conversation. Sometimes you need to suggest that you check back in a few hours or the next day to discuss solutions depending on how the other person is feeling. If you suggest doing this, you need to follow through, no matter how uncomfortable it feels – trust me, it's far more uncomfortable to leave things hanging.

When you ask for input, listen to the other person's perspective and ideas. Then you can share your own ideas but only after you have really listened. Often people will come up with far better solutions than you will and most importantly, they will be committed to them because they suggested them.

D stands for **Desired Outcome**. You want to make sure you are both clear on a desired outcome. It's valuable to come up with this together as you are both invested in it and it doesn't feel like one person telling the other what to do (yes, this works well even when you are a manager speaking to an employee). In the example from earlier, the desired outcome may be that you both feel included in conversations or work events. Usually the **Desired Outcome** will grow organically from having listened well to one another.

After you have both agreed to the desired outcome, set a time to follow up and see how things are going. This gives you an opportunity to check in. If things are still off track, you can discuss other solutions. If things are on track, you can focus on what's working and build on that.

This feedback model is not just for dealing with difficult situations or people. It is so important that we make the time to point out what is working really well in our relationships – taking two minutes to share a specific action someone took and the positive impact it had on you will go miles towards building strong relationships, both at home and at work.

I encourage you to give feedback as often as possible, both positive and constructive feedback. The more comfortable and practiced you become, the easier it is to do. Often, when we let someone know about their behaviour and its impact on us, that is enough for them to make a change. Other times, they won't change no matter what we say or do. But then you've done your best, you have taken action to reduce your stress. If you've given someone feedback and things haven't changed, you can focus on how you respond to their behaviour because that's what you can control. And your response has to be to shrug it off and move on, otherwise you're creating way too much stress for yourself.

Before you give any feedback, you need to consider the timing and how the other person is feeling. Ask when would be a good time to talk, and make sure you're creating the best dynamics possible for a productive conversation.

I strongly encourage you to give people feedback when there are challenges in your relationship. You may not see any results, but you will have done what you can to address the issue. You can't change another person, you can only change yourself. On that note, I also encourage you to ask for feedback. It's possible that the person who is your biggest nightmare also finds you quite difficult. If you can find the courage to have a feedback conversation, you may both learn something that will help you grow.

If you do decide to ask for feedback, follow the same model as giving feedback. Ask for feedback on a **Specific action** or behaviour (or recent interaction) and ask the person to share what the **Impact** was on them. Sometimes asking for feedback is all that is needed to shift the dynamics. When we show that we are willing to make changes in our own behaviour to improve the relationship, others will often appreciate this and feel more open to making changes themselves. If you ask someone how you can have a stronger working relationship or communicate better with them, they may give you useful information that helps you adapt your actions and behaviour. Asking someone for feedback is a great place to start, because our behaviour and our reaction is the only aspect of any relationship that we can control. We can give other people feedback but we can't control what they do with it.

We are hardwired to get defensive when we receive feedback - it hurts because we have a fundamental need to be accepted and we perceive feedback as a threat. When giving feedback, be prepared for a defensive reaction. When this happens, acknowledge that it's hard to hear difficult feedback, and express that you appreciate the person listening to your concerns. When someone is giving you feedback and you feel tempted to defend yourself, don't. Thank the person for sharing their feedback as you know it takes courage. Then see what you can learn from the feedback they have offered you.

When I'm assessing whether I should give another person difficult feedback, I consider how much energy I'm putting into the issue. Is it keeping me awake at night? Is it impacting our working relationship? Is it impacting the work we are doing? Am I talking to a coach or trusted friend about it? If so, I always choose to give feedback. Giving feedback is an action I can take to resolve the situation that is bothering me. I give feedback and then let go of the outcome. I hope that the other person will change, but I can't control that. All I can control is what I do and when I've had the courage to have a difficult feedback conversation, I feel good because I've taken action.

We encounter all kinds of challenging situations and personalities at work and in our lives. If we want to reduce our stress, we have to make the choice to be courageous, take action and have difficult conversations to address the challenges we are facing.

3. Quit taking things personally

Believe it or not, most of the things that happen at work aren't about you. There are big organizational systems at play that impact many elements of your workplace, but they aren't about you.

There are some people who think that management sits around in a room and thinks up ways to make their lives miserable. But that's not reality. Management may come up with some ideas that don't work or implement some ridiculous systems, but the intent is always to improve some aspect of the organization, not to make employees' lives miserable. That may be an unfortunate side effect and that's when it's important to give feedback.

Many workplace changes aren't handled well, and many large organizational systems do not always serve employees, but it's not personal. It's about the organization. If you feel like a change has been made specifically with you in mind, go and ask for clarification to understand why the decision was made and the impact it will have on you.

In addition to organizational issues, we often take other people's behaviour personally. Don't take what others say and do personally. 90% of the time it's not about you, it's about them. Think carefully and see if there's anything you may have done to contribute to the situation or dynamic. If there is, do something to rectify the situation then let it go. If there isn't, don't take it personally. Recognise that people engage in a lot of unhealthy behaviours, but most of the time it's not about you.

I can't tell you the number of workplace conflicts I've facilitated because people are taking things personally. I once worked with a team who was in conflict because their manager was quite controlling She was a perfectionist and did things herself because she believed no one else could possibly do them to the same standard that she did. How do you think her team responded? Did they say, "Oh, that's just her, being a perfectionist, nothing to do with me?" No, they said, "she doesn't trust me," and "she is holding a grudge from that time I screwed up that project three years ago," and "she thinks my work is inferior," and "I think she's planning to fire me." In short, they made up stories, stories in which they were the main character. It's not about you. Don't get caught up in other people's drama.

If there's something that's bothering you, go and seek clarification, ask for feedback, share your feedback, tell the person about the impact of their behaviour, and discuss a way to work it out. A great way to start this conversation is "I know I'm probably totally off-base here….", or "I'm really confused about what's going on and rather than make up stories in my head, I thought I'd come talk to you."

Most of us will have to work with difficult people, even ones who will occasionally be impossible. I know it, I've lived it and I've coached people through it. I'm not saying it's going to be all roses from here on in, but you will significantly reduce your stress if you don't take their behaviour personally.

Your job is to figure out how you can work with a difficult person, and get your work done. You don't have to be best friends, but you do need to have a good, professional working relationship. Be the bigger person. When you stop engaging in their drama, the dynamics will shift and you can be far more rational when responding to them. Instead of raging at or about the difficult person that you work with, consider them a teacher. They are teaching you to manage your reactions and to be professional in spite of trying circumstances.

You can't control what other people do or how the organization operates but you can control how you respond to it. When you can respond to stressful situations in a professional way and don't take things personally, you significantly decrease your stress.

4. Take Personal Responsibility

90% of what people do or say isn't about you, it's about them. This applies to you too. 90% of your behaviour is about you. Your reactions to people, situations and stressors at work are about you, not about them. I can walk into two different people's offices, deliver exactly the same hard-to-hear message and get two completely different responses. One person might get angry, defensive or start blaming others; the other may go quiet and ask questions to get a better understanding about what their role is and how they can improve things. Same situation, same message, totally different responses.

What is your natural response in difficult situations? How can you reflect and take personal responsibility when needed? I suggest you ask yourself the same questions to help you take personal responsibility rather than blaming others for the situation.

Why is this so upsetting for me? This helps you identify what you're feeling and why.

How did I contribute to this? This helps you identify the specific things you did that contributed to the situation.

What can I learn from this? When you focus on learning from the situation, you can focus on growing rather than stressing out.

What can I do about this situation? This helps you focus on specific solutions and strategies.

What can I do differently next time? This helps you identify the specific things you will change in a similar situation in the future.

We have to take responsibility for ourselves. It's not up to anyone else to make us happy, productive and engaged at work. It's up to us. Marshall Goldsmith, a phenomenal leadership coach and author encourages us to ask the following questions when we think about our own engagement at work.

1. Did I do my best to increase my happiness?

2. Did I do my best to find meaning?
3. Did I do my best to be engaged?
4. Did I do my best to build positive relationships?
5. Did I do my best to set clear goals?
6. Did I do my best to make progress toward goal achievement?[4]

I love this approach because too often we think it's the organization's responsibility to make us happy. I have worked in many wonderful organizations that are doing everything right, which results in 95% of their staff being highly engaged, productive employees. The employees that aren't engaged are not taking any personal responsibility for how they show up and the impact they have on others.

What behaviours do you engage in at work that aren't healthy? Here are a few that I've seen.

➤ Slacking off and hoping that no one will call you on it
➤ Gossiping about others at work or listening to gossip
➤ When you have a challenge with someone at work, you don't talk to them about it, you talk to everyone else
➤ Getting into conflict repeatedly
➤ Wanting things done your way because you know best
➤ Thinking everyone you work with is an idiot and you've never made a mistake or caused a problem
➤ Getting into cliques and leaving some people 'out'

---

4 http://www.marshallgoldsmith.com/articles/6-questions-that-will-set-you-up-to-be-super-successful/

- ➢ Refusing to speak to some people
- ➢ Speaking disrespectfully to others, either because of their role, or a previous relationship challenge
- ➢ Not speaking up when you disagree with a work direction or idea but then talking non-stop about it to everyone who will listen, trying to get them on your side
- ➢ Not getting over a conflict from the past – treating someone badly because of a previous interaction
- ➢ Not getting over a difficult work situation in the past and hating 'management' for what has happened (regardless of how long ago it happened or who was in management then)
- ➢ Not being open to new ideas
- ➢ Being overly critical and negative
- ➢ Feeling complacent and uninterested in doing good work or building good relationships
- ➢ Focusing on what won't work and your frustrations, rather than solutions
- ➢ Blaming others rather than looking for solutions or how you may have contributed to the problem
- ➢ Keeping information to yourself – not sharing information because information is power
- ➢ Being judgmental of others, making up stories about how and why they are behaving certain ways rather than talking to them and listening with an open mind

We all engage in some of these behaviours some of the time. We are human. And we are influenced by our workplace culture. You might be a person who never gossips but everyone at work is gossiping so you join the conversation too. You might be the hardest worker ever but you work with a bunch of slackers, so you start slacking too.

We aren't perfect. But we can strive to be better. We have to start paying attention to how we behave at work and recognise the impact we are having. Then we can make choices. Sometimes we aren't even aware of what we are doing or the impact it's having. If you engage in negative behaviour, you're contributing to a negative workplace culture. If you engage in positive behaviour, you're contributing to a positive workplace culture. Slowly but surely, we can start to eliminate some of our negative behaviours and replace them with positive behaviours. Take a good long look at your behaviour and attitude. Ask yourself, am I having a positive impact at work or a negative impact? Be honest with yourself and work to change any negative behaviours you're engaging in. When you're focusing on being positive and engaged, you'll feel so much better about yourself and you'll enjoy work a lot more. Give it a try, it can't hurt.

Taking personal responsibility means that you genuinely try to make things work - you focus on what you can do in a situation rather than blaming others and you take action. When you take personal responsibility for your attitude and behaviours, your stress decreases significantly, because you create less stress in your life.

5. Own Your Mistakes

I once had an interview for my dream job. But somehow I wrote down the date wrong, and thought the interview was on a Wednesday. When the interviewers called on Tuesday at 1:10 to ask where I was, I couldn't believe what I had done. I apologized profusely and offered to rush over to their office, but it was too late since they had the next candidate arriving soon. I was so upset with myself as this was my dream job, I called a friend and talked it through. I decided to put on my suit, buy a box of chocolates and a card, and take it to the office. I didn't meet with any of them, but I delivered my gifts of apology. That night, they called me to set up an interview the next week. Amazingly, I got the job. They told me later that they were impressed that I was able to acknowledge and apologize for a mistake.

We are all going to screw up but rather than stressing out endlessly about our screw-ups, we have to focus on how we can rectify the situation. I suggest you ask yourself the same questions when you've made a mistake:

Why is this so upsetting for me? This helps you identify what you're feeling and why.

How did I contribute to this? This helps you identify the specific things you did that contributed to the situation.

What can I learn from this? When you focus on learning from the situation, you can focus on growing rather than stressing out.

What can I do about this situation? This helps you focus on specific solutions and strategies.

What can I do differently next time? This helps you identify the specific things you will change in a similar situation in the future.

Once you've apologized and made amends, and learned from the situation, you need to let it go and move on. Rather than dwelling on it, put it in the past and focus on what you can do better in the present. Our mind can only hold one thought at a time and we want to focus it on a productive thought, rather than a negative one that brings us down.

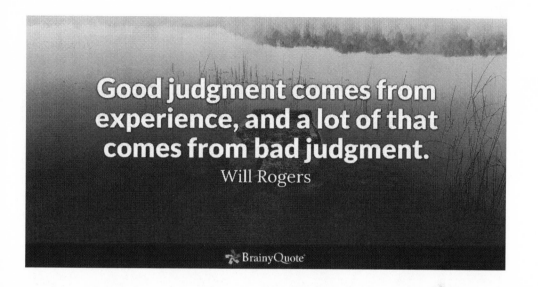

Good judgment comes from experience, and a lot of that comes from bad judgment.
Will Rogers
BrainyQuote

When we can see mistakes as opportunities to learn, we have a completely different attitude. I once had a client whose employee made a mistake that cost the company $250,000. My client asked his employee what he learned from the situation; when he heard all the growth and learning that had taken place, he said, "Well, that was my $250,000 investment in you and your learning." He let it go and moved on. I'm sure that if the employee hadn't acknowledged his mistake and what he learned from it, the outcome would have been much different.

We all make mistakes - no-one can be operating at 100% all of the time. Cut yourself some slack. Let go of worrying about what's happened in the past, focus on what you can learn, and how you can move on. People will respect you far more if you are honest and acknowledge your mistakes than if you try to cover them up, blame others, or pretend they didn't happen. When we genuinely appreciate the learning that comes from our mistakes, we reduce our stress significantly.

6. Own Your Choices

Recognize you are making a choice to be at your job. Seriously. Every day, you are making a choice to be there. If you hate your stressful job but you keep choosing it, you need to question your choices. There are other jobs. Start looking. Maybe they won't pay as well or the benefits won't be as good or there won't be as much vacation time but if they make you happier, giving those things up is worth it. Nothing is worth being miserable for 8 hours a day every day. Workplace stress takes a significant toll on our health, our relationships and our life. We need to get it under control.

If you have done your best to be professional and positive and you realise that you are working in a toxic workplace, with no end in sight, then I strongly encourage you to look for another job. A toxic workplace is very different than being in a regular workplace. A regular workplace has challenges, but people are genuinely trying to make things work. A toxic work environment includes but is not limited to employees consistently not being respected by management; unreasonable demands on time and effort; a culture of negativity and gossip; a fear-based management style; overwhelming anxiety; and, no room to question ideas or contribute. Working in this kind of environment is not worth the toll it takes on you. If this is your workplace, find another job.

I once had a client who realised that he was never going to be happy in the organization he worked in and he needed to find a job that was a better fit for him. He ended up finding a job that looked great but there was a significant pay cut. He decided to go for it and after a few months in the new job, he said he'd taken a $20,000 decrease in pay and a 200% increase in happiness. Three years later, he had worked his way up in the new organization and was making more money than he had in his previous role. It takes courage and faith that things will work out but it's worth it to find work that feels right for you.

We all look for three fundamental needs to be met by work – survival, belonging, and contribution. Work helps us pay the rent and put food on the table; gives us a sense of belonging and connection, and provides us with the opportunity to contribute our gifts and strengths. If you don't get these things from your workplace, it can be very stressful. Sometimes there is a values mismatch, the work culture is unhealthy, or you aren't working in an area of your strength. If this is the case for you, I encourage you to look for a job that meets your fundamental needs – financial stability, a sense of belonging and the ability to contribute your strengths and natural talents.

If you choose to stay in your job, learn to appreciate what's good about it. Maybe it's not your dream job but it gives you time for your other passions. Maybe you really love the people you work with, or the benefits are fantastic. Maybe you're learning a lot. You've made the choice to be there so you may as well make the choice to make it a worthwhile and enjoyable experience.

If you realise you need to make different choices, don't contribute to a negative workplace by focusing on what's not working and complaining about things you can't change. Continue to be professional and focus on what you appreciate about your job while looking around for a job that's a better fit for you.

When we focus on what is good and what works in our lives, we draw more of that to us. When we focus on what's negative and isn't working, we draw more of that to us. Even if there is just one little thing that is good about your job, spend your time focusing on it. It makes you feel better; it helps you appreciate what works; and, focusing on the good stuff will create more positive energy in your life.

7. Set boundaries

Setting boundaries is a key strategy in reducing our stress. We need to recognise what's realistic for us, stop trying to please everyone else, and pushing ourselves to be overachievers. We have to learn to say no. It costs us too much not to.

Workloads have become overwhelming. I see so many people who are extremely stressed out by all that work demands of them, not to mention their responsibilities to family. We need to prioritize our work, figure out what's most important, and focus on completing and delivering the important work. If you don't have clarity on this, use your manager as a resource – ask them what they see as the most important deliverable on your plate and then focus on that. One project well done is far better than three projects half-done, and an employee off on stress leave. We need to learn to prioritize, to say no, and to set reasonable expectations.

It is difficult to reduce our workloads and start saying no but we have to - otherwise we become far less productive. Research has shown time and again that the extra hours you are putting in aren't making you more productive. They're making you less productive.

> Research found that employee output falls sharply after a 50-hour work-week, and falls off a cliff after 55 hours—so much so that someone who puts in 70 hours produces nothing more with those extra 15 hours, according to a study published by John Pencavel of Stanford University[5].

We can't do it all. When we try, everything suffers – the work, our physical and mental health, our relationships, and our energy for life.

Get really clear on your priorities and be prepared to defend and explain your decisions. We need to think things through, set boundaries, and explain our decisions to those we work with. Learn

5   https://www.cnbc.com/2015/01/26/working-more-than-50-hours-makes-you-less-productive.html

to say "If I take this on, something has to come off my plate or I'll be doing substandard work" or "If I prioritize this, it means I need to delay the timelines for the other project" or "I will be leaving at 5 today to catch my son's soccer game because it's important to me." You have to set good boundaries in order to set yourself up for success.

Too often I take on too much work because I love helping people and I genuinely enjoy my work. But I don't set myself up for success when I say yes to too much work. I prevent myself from overcommitting by reminding myself that when I'm stretched too thin, I'm not doing my best work. When I say yes to more work, that means I'm saying no to other elements of my life or work, such as writing or time with my kids.

Get clear on what your priorities are - at work and at home - and then filter every decision you make through those priorities. My number one priority is my family. I took a huge leap three years ago, after my second child was born, to move from being an employee to working as a consultant. It turned out very well, allowing me to earn more and balance doing the work I love with being able to spend more time with my kids. It was terrifying to quit my job and take the leap but it was so worth it. Because I can set my own schedule, I'm able to drop my kids off at school and daycare and pick them up, I schedule my work around their field trips and concerts and special events and I'm able to spend my summers with my kids.

However, the boundary challenge didn't go away. I still need to clarify and prioritize my work and say no to taking on too much. I have often struggled with setting boundaries and I've had to keep learning how to do it. To deal with too much work, I recently hired another facilitator so I can keep a good life-work balance. Our challenges don't disappear, they follow us wherever we go until we resolve them.

When we put boundaries in place to manage the demands on us, we are able to perform better, have more energy for our work, and have good attention for our colleagues, our friends and family members. Know your limit and work within it. Take your lunch and coffee breaks, take your vacation time. When you take time for yourself to recharge, you will feel better, be less stressed and get more done. When you notice your good motivational 'eustress' becoming stress, identify what you need to change and take action. It will benefit you, your company and your family.

Setting boundaries includes disconnecting. It's far too easy to connect to work after hours and too many of us do it. It's not helping us. Research has shown that when we disconnect, we return recharged and we are far more productive. We are becoming addicted to our phones but we need to put down our phones and spend time relaxing and re-energizing.

Having good boundaries means that when you aren't at work, you don't work. Too many of us check and send emails when we should be spending that time with our loved ones. Not only does taking a break from your email help you strengthen your personal relationships, it also increases your productivity. Many companies are recognising the value of this and forcing employees to disconnect.

Volkswagen programs employee's phones to switch off work emails automatically from 6 pm to 7 am. A study by researchers from the University of California, Irivine and the US Army found that avoiding your inbox – taking an email vacation – reduces stress and allows you to focus more. When an entire company 'Learning as Leadership' forbid email for an entire week, [they] experienced a more focused and productive energy...the decrease in stress from one day to the next was palpable. So was [the] increase in energy."[6]

Leading edge companies know that forcing their employees to disconnect is good for productivity as well as employee health. Follow their lead and disconnect. Setting boundaries with work allows us to have time and energy for what's most important, our relationships. Research coming out of Harvard's recent 75 year-long study on what makes a good life argues that good relationships lead to a long and fulfilling life[7]. Most of us know this intuitively but can get sucked in to work and forget about what gives us true happiness and fulfilment.

Many of the people I coach struggle with life-work balance. That's not a typo....I write it that way deliberately to remind us that life should come first. At the end of our lives, we are not remembered for the work we have done but for the people we have touched. I have one client who is constantly connected to work and to his phone. And with good reason - he is actually saving lives. Most people can draw the line with work and justify taking personal time by saying "Well, we're not saving lives"; this is not his case, so I understand

6 Thrive, Arianna Huffington, P. 66
7 https://www.health.harvard.edu/blog/the-secret-to-happiness-heres-some-advice-from-the-longest-running-study-on-happiness-2017100512543

why it is hard for him to disconnect. I can also see that with such a high-pressure profession, it is more important than ever for him to disconnect.

He recently told me a story about a time in his early twenties when he had to choose between a job and the girl that he was in love with. He told me with pride that he chose the girl, and they have been married for almost 30 years. A lifetime ago, he made the grand romantic gesture and it was the right choice. As we talked more about his need for balance, it became clear that over time, in little choices he made, in the competing demands of work and life, he wasn't always able to choose the girl.

This is how it happens; we lose perspective bit by bit and work begins to creep into the cherished spaces reserved for family and friends. When work takes priority, it can become difficult to reconnect to the people we have been putting aside. Different versions of this can happen to any of us. But it's crucial to make a conscious choice to reconnect with the people who are most important to us. It may take an apology and redeeming ourselves through genuine and heartfelt actions to show our loved ones that they are important to us but it's worth the effort.

At the end of the day, it is those that we love who matter most in the world. We often realize this when we lose them, and we yearn for just a minute more with them. I share some of my own insights about this experience in my book, 9 Strategies for Dealing with the Difficult Stuff. Don't wait until someone is gone to comprehend the value of your time with them. Make space for them now – be deliberate about this. Whatever stage of life you are at, whatever is going on at work, choose the girl, the boy, the child, or the friend; whoever is competing with the job, choose them. Our time and attention is the biggest gift that we can give anyone; it's the way that we can show people that we love them.

Work gives us many things but not everything. When you find yourself slipping into focusing more on work, take a step back and remember that no one at your funeral will speak of what a good employee you were - they will speak of what a good parent you were, what a good friend you were, and what a good spouse you were, because you made the time for your cherished relationships.

Steal back your time from work, go home early, put the phone away. Ask the people you love to spend time with you – time when you disconnect from everything but them. Give them your full attention. Put the time and the effort into having quality relationships. It's the most important thing you can do. Set good boundaries so you can get good work done, and at the end of the day, you'll have time and energy to spend with those you love.

8. Build positive relationships

We spend 8 hours every day with our colleagues. That's usually more time than we spend with the person we've chosen to marry, our friends, or our family. Why would you not want to have pleasant and professional relationships with these people?

I work with a lot of teams that are stressed out, with high workloads and big demands, but their number one stressor seems to be interpersonal relationships. It's tough dealing with other people all day long, especially when they aren't people you would have chosen to spend a significant part of your life with. We need to find ways to manage all our relationships professionally and focus on building strong relationships with the people we do enjoy.

Research has proven repeatedly that good working relationships lead to higher productivity and more workplace satisfaction. A study done by MIT of IBM employees found that the more socially connected the IBM employees were, the better they performed.[8]

In a recent study of workplace dynamics reported in the Harvard Business Review, researchers "found that … having a lot of coworkers who eventually developed into friends, significantly increased employees' performance, as judged by their supervisor. One possible reason for this was people seeking advice. If you have friends in the company, it's far easier to ask for help without fearing you'll be judged a poor performer. In addition, having friends in the company, especially if they work in other departments, gives you access to information through informal networks you might not otherwise get. Another reason might be morale: Employees with close friends at work reported being in a good mood more often, which could spill over into positive effects on the work being performed."[9]

Too often at work we are focused on getting work done but if we also focus on building strong relationships, we will be more productive, engaged and successful at work.

8 (The Happiness Advantage, Shawn Achor, p. 186,)
9 https://hbr.org/2017/05/work-friends-make-us-more-productive-except-when-they-stress-us-out

I love people - I enjoy getting to know and understand them, cracking jokes and having fun together. I'm genuinely interested in people but I never brought my social side fully into work because I thought it was unprofessional. Then I did my masters in leadership, and discovered all the research that shows the value of building positive relationships with people at work. I was encouraged by my profs to be as social and friendly in my workplace as I was in the rest of my life. I started asking about people's weekends, learning more about their lives, and making connections. I shared more about myself and my life, and this invited others to open up too. I developed close friends. Work didn't suffer for those ten minutes that were spent chatting in the morning or the extra fifteen minutes taken on a lunch break as we laughed about a meeting that went sideways or a long coffee that was taken just to listen to each other. No, ...we connected and our work life flourished because of it.

We are social beings. We need to connect with other people. Gallup, a company that conducts research on employee engagement and organizational effectiveness has designed twelve questions to help assess employee engagement.

Here are three of them:

- ✓ Does your supervisor, or someone at work, seem to care about you as a person?
- ✓ Is there someone at work who encourages your development?
- ✓ Do you have a best friend at work?

Having good friends and caring relationships at work gives us a sense of belonging and connection. Research has shown that we will stay at a workplace longer and work harder when we have friends at work. Friends make everything more enjoyable, even work.

I hear so many people say that they don't want to be friends with people they work with, that they don't even like them. Fair enough, that's your choice. Just know that it will increase your stress to have more difficult working relationships. And it will decrease your stress to build friendships at work. You are making a choice. Sometimes we forget that. At the bare minimum, you need to be professional and respectful - talking to your colleagues in a respectful tone, engaging in discussions with an open mind, and working effectively together. If you do choose to build stronger connections at work, take the time to ask people about themselves and their lives. I've been consistently surprised when I get to know people better – everyone has an interesting story. You'll often find common ground, new respect and compassion for your co-workers by getting to know people on a personal level. Open up and share something about yourself and people will often respond in kind. Be kind to people - find things you appreciate about them and give them positive feedback. It'll have a great impact on them, on their productivity and on your working relationship.

I have coached many people who have been frustrated by difficult co-workers and yet are not willing to make changes to their relationship. The longer I coached them, the more apparent it became that they were the source of their own stress. By changing their attitude and behaviour to be more respectful and professional, and maybe even a bit friendlier, the entire workplace dynamics shifted. It's up to you. Building positive relationships at work can increase your productivity and your enjoyment and significantly reduce your stress.

> "People will forget what you said, people will forget what you did but they will never forget how you made them feel" – Maya Angelou

9. Shift your mind-set

You are the only person that can control the amount of stress you have because your stress levels are a direct result of how you react to a situation. We often don't think of this as a strategy to manage stress but when we can change our reaction to stressful events, we can significantly reduce our stress. Maybe someone at work says something really unprofessional, upsetting or irritating. You have choices in how you react. You can shrug your shoulders, say "Hmm, he must be having a bad day," and move on, or you can get upset, or you can vent with everyone in the office about it, or dwell on it as you're falling asleep. You can let it go, or you can stress yourself out, or – if it warrants it - you can also choose to address the situation by talking directly to the person in order to let them know how their comment or behaviour impacted you. Same event, many different responses.

Changing our attitude can help us shift from someone who is highly stressed to someone who is relaxed and easy going. Think back to a work situation that you found really stressful a year ago. Chances are you can't get yourself worked up about it now. We need to put things in perspective as they are happening.

5 BY 5 RULE

If it's not going to matter in 5 years, don't spend more than 5 minutes being upset by it.

Putting things in perspective is an excellent way to shift our mind-set. Years ago my husband worked for a manager who provided some excellent perspective for him. My husband was working as an engineer at a company that designed and installed industrial boilers. He was taking time off to be with his father, who just had an aneurysm, when his sister became suddenly ill and died. It was his first job after graduating from university; he had only been working there a matter of months, and he was working on large proposals with short deadlines. He was worried about all the time he had to take off from work. When he spoke to his boss about his concerns, his boss responded by saying, "It's only boilers."

This man had perspective. He knew what was most important in life, and it wasn't work – it was to be with the people you love when they need you. Time is precious, and it becomes more precious when our loved ones need us. I'm so grateful that my husband's boss had the wisdom to offer him this perspective and gave him the freedom to spend time with his family when they needed him.

Often much of our stress comes not from the event itself but from our feeling that it shouldn't have happened. We can increase our stress and suffering a great deal by not accepting reality. We can waste countless hours and precious energy being upset that something happened or is happening, rather than accepting reality. It's reality, it is happening. The more time we spend being upset about reality rather than accepting it, the more stressed out we are. A client of mine was fired from her job. She had no idea it was coming, was deeply upset and felt it was unfair. She caused herself far more stress by focusing on what should have happened rather than what did happen. Her manager should have talked to her, they should have offered her coaching, her last performance review was a good one, they should have told her there were issues.

While all those things may have been true, there was nothing she could do about any of them. She needed to stop thinking about what should have happened and start accepting what did happen. We talked through what she could do to accept that she had been fired. She realised that she needed to fully experience and then let go of her feelings. She recognised that she had been stuck in stress and anger about something she couldn't change. We talked through all the ways she felt – betrayed, manipulated, unfairly treated, worried about her financial situation and reputation. She felt her feelings, talked them through and then was able to let them go because she recognised that she couldn't change what had happened. She then turned her focus to what she could control – learning from the situation and finding a new job. It was important for her to be able to feel everything and take some time to lick her wounds and then move on and focus on solutions.

Stress is a given - when we can approach it with a different attitude and a bit of perspective, it helps us reduce it. Don't waste your energy - make a conscious effort to let go of the things you have absolutely no control over. Turn your focus to what you can control and how you can contribute to decreasing the stress in your life. When you shift your mindset, you can significantly reduce your stress.

CONCLUSION

Stressful events are a natural part of life. The more skilled we get at responding to them, the better our lives will be. We all juggle multiple commitments and responsibilities, both at work and in life. Stress is not going to go away and I hope that the strategies I've shared here will be helpful to you in managing your stress so you can reduce its impact on you. Remember to choose one or two that you think would help you and start using them. Changing our mindset and behaviour takes time but the sooner you use these strategies, the sooner you'll see positive results.

None of the strategies I've shared here are rocket science – many of you have probably read and heard about them before. What I've found that makes the difference in whether we use them or not is courage. Do we have the courage to take action, have that difficult conversation, take personal responsibility? Often our fear stops us. We let fear hold us back but then we create more stress in our lives by not dealing with our challenges. Pick a strategy, start small and go for it. Reducing your stress will lead to a healthier, happier life and that's worth pushing through your fear.

When you're feeling more relaxed and able to cope with the many demands of life, life feels better. Reducing your stress will give you more energy for the people that you love and the things you really enjoy in life. Your health, relationships and work will all benefit when you reduce your stress.

My mission in life is to support people to have good lives – more meaningful, more connected, more relaxed, and happier lives no matter what challenging or stressful experiences we may have. I hope that the strategies I've shared here will help you to reduce your stress and enjoy life more. Let me know how it goes – I'd love to hear about it. You can email me at Stephanie@stephanieberryman.com or post your comment on my facebook page at https://www.facebook.com/stephanieberrymanauthor/ or leave me a review on Amazon.

If you'd like more strategies and ideas about how to live a good life in spite of the stress and challenges we face every day, come join me at www.stephanieberryman.com. Or follow me on Medium https://medium.com/@stephanieberry. You'll receive my free e-book *The Good Life Manifesto* about what makes a really good life. I also have a few other titles available with completely different strategies for just $0.99 on Amazon – 9 strategies for dealing with stress and 9 strategies for dealing with the difficult stuff . If you'd like to learn more about my leadership consulting and coaching, please visit my website – www.managetoengage.com. Thanks for taking the time to read my book – I wish for you a good life, one with healthy levels of stress that continue to engage and inspire you.

Appendix A:

Lifestyle Strategies (generously shared by my readers, colleagues, clients and friends)

Sometimes you have to turn everything off and take a nap.

—**Kami Boley**

Don't skip your breaks.

—**Nicole Mackey**

Many years ago I had a high stress job managing a lot of legal deadlines & never-ending paperwork, and worked in a cubicle with no privacy and lots of interruptions. I installed a 'closed door' in my cube by stringing a length of yarn across the opening with a paper sign hanging right in the middle of it that said "Do Not Disturb - Back at (insert sticky note with time)" to give myself blocks of uninterrupted time to focus. Simple solution... but it worked!!

—**Kathleen Koprowski**

Remember that, in the long run, it's just a job. It is not worth ruining your health or relationships. After you leave, the company will continue thriving without you.

—**Cindi Franer**

I used to go to lunch, go to sonic and sit in the car to give myself space and to get myself composed enough for the afternoon.

—**Loretta Vise Gjeltema**

Schedule Time for Work. Put your work hours on your calendar. When it's time to stop and go home, stop and go home. Then home time is home time and work time is work time. Control your time, so it doesn't control you.

—**Shayne Seymour** - www.independentlyhappy.com

Get grounded before you go in. Assure clarity on expectations. Be able to know that you nailed it today. Don't let distractions, or other people's agendas, keep you from the clear goals. Then, keep an eye out for whom you can encourage. If possible, arrive early to get settled before the day begins.

—**Kevin Cunningham,** www.EncourageAndEquip.com

I teach my students this process when they are overwhelmed (something I learned at work running a nonprofit one year): Take a deep breath, say "I can do this". Prioritize tasks, take action on task 1, and repeat. One thing at a time, ten minute blocks, keeping the bigger "why" in mind and releasing the expectation of perfection.

—**Sue Larkins Weems**

Try not to rush through your work. Quality is better than quantity. Know that your integrity is valuable. Less stress is far better than more money. Keep work at work. Have clear boundaries...distinct work times, family time and fun time.

—**Rachel Larkin**

One of the best ways to reduce stress is to be mindful and honest about what you really can control and what is outside of your control. So many times we let ourselves get all worked up about events, deadlines, nasty co-workers, office politics and more when 90% is beyond our control. About the only thing we really, truly have full control over is how we respond to what happens. If we can purposefully respond with confidence, competence, compassion, and respect for both our personal dignity and the dignity of others, then we can rest assured we've done all we can do.

—**Susan Scott**

The hospital I work at has fancy massage chairs in their break rooms. It even massages our feet. They really care about their nurses there. Happy Nurse, Happy Patients! -Vagabond RN.

—**Kayla Guzman**

As someone with a short commute I say "take the long way home." Make sure you disconnect and leave it at the office. Give yourself a moment to just breathe and refocus on home.

—**Maxwell Davidson**

Live a balanced life. I was so stressed at work I was tired all the time and did nothing else. A mix of different activities and seeing friends keeps me sane. Stops me dwelling on any one thing.

—**Fiona Bruff**

When I get stressed, I take a breath break. I stop what I'm doing and take one slow full breath in while focusing on my side ribs expanding, then slowly exhale while noticing the side ribs coming back toward each other, kind of like an accordion. It's quick and easy, it calms me down, and it works anytime, anywhere!

—**Kris Loomis**

I run. It gives me something else to focus on while also providing some time away from the situations that are adding to the stress. Just put my ear buds in and go!

—**Brandon Weldy**

I pray. Talking to God always calms me down.

—**Jan Cox**

I do a simple mindfulness exercise. I take deep breaths for a minute, feeling the breath come in through my nose, focusing on the cold air going down my throat, feeling my lungs fill up, and then exhale.

—**Anders Ferrer**

Take advantage of your break and lunch times. You don't have to do the same thing every time you take a break. Some breaks can be a time for prayer/meditation. Other times, you can walk around the building or around the outside of the building if it's nice outside. You can also work on your book/blog/other side project.

Also, have one major activity/group outside of work that helps you and helps others. This will help you to remember that there's life outside of work. Volunteer. Join one of your church's groups or help with church services. Start a side gig (writing a book, blogging). Join a local group where members share the same hobby, side gig, or other interests.

—**Maya Spikes**

Understand quickly how to maintain your own personal passions outside of work because having both will make both better for everyone. Maximize free time. If you want to escape a job then your Work is never done until you do. Devote real time to stress reduction, you often can't undo stress with thinking so focus on positive actions and do what makes you feel good inside!

—**Greg Narayan**

It depends on what level/type of stress you're talking about. If it's the stress of a deadline, I listen to relaxing music (classical for me). If it's a routine task that has gone haywire, I switch tasks for a while and come back with a fresh perspective that often resolves the problem. If it's a stressful work environment (coworkers, clients, etc.), I try to avoid the drama as much as possible and concentrate on accomplishing my goals/projects.

—Dalene Bickel

Go for a run

—JT Woodwalker

Leave the office at lunch time, change into the flat shoes you keep under your desk, leave your phone in your purse, and walk for 20 minutes

—Meredith Sargent

Don't work when you're not at work

—Kristi Fairholm-Mader

Take breaks. Always eat. Go for walks. Deep breaths. Drink plenty of water.

—Marwan Talian

The last place I worked the owner brought in his golden retriever everyday, she would make her rounds and visit everyone.

—Devon Olafson

Make a short list of the "must get done today" things that you can't ignore. Make it brief. Accept that you can't and won't get it all done. Accept that the list must be flexible. And don't be afraid to ask for help. "Many hands make light work!"

—**Marjorie Millman**

Eating healthy snacks (veggies & fruits), drinking water, and soothing music helps. Teachers don't get to leave the classroom some days so I work it into my classroom management plan. We do some deep breathing and relaxation in the afternoon and then some energizers. Lighting, calm colours, plants and other aesthetics are helpful for students and myself included.

—**Tammy Obey**

If it's terrible, quit. If you can't quit - make space for connection and laughter with colleagues. Share wins and laugh about what's beyond your control.

—**Kim Mahood Walters**

In my office, we say "Don't get it right, get it written." Translation: identify what "Good Enough" means and what costs (personal or organisational) are added to go beyond that. Even Olympic athletes don't train at 100% every single time.

—**Allan Tyler**

Bring in treats to the office now and then.

—Jenny Nash

Don't evangelize about your self-care while at work, but don't try to hide it or downplay it either. Be forthright about how you're taking a few moments or setting boundaries. One of my best moments at work was when, after having just worked 12 hours, my boss texted me at home to ask if I was currently taking notes on what had just happened in my work day "while the details were fresh". I was tempted to not reply or to lie and say I was. But instead I responded that I was now at home with my family and that I'd pick it up tomorrow at 9am. She wrote back "lol. Ok. So am I and so will I."

—John Woods

My mantra on those 'omg' or 'wtf' kinda days was "deepen the breath, still the mind"

—Anni Holtby

I used different approaches for my stress vs my team's stress... employee fun days and early Friday lunch ... whirly ball and laser tag was great for getting rid of social and hierarchical stress... my own stress... well... I ended up quitting and going into fine art.

—Kris Bovenizer

I find it impossible to take deep breaths or meditate or other mindful things when I'm really stressed. I have to move to calm myself - a long walk outside is ideal, but if I can't get outside, I just jog in place in front of an open window, or dance around to some loud music. The cardio FORCES you to breathe, and then the endorphins come along ... It's backwards, I know, but if I change how I feel physically, I change my emotional state as well.

— **Kay Bolden**

Here are a few things that I do: Regular physical activity (before and after work), practice mindfulness when possible (lunch time, walking to meetings etc.), focus on issues and not emotions behind the issues, keep things in perspective, focus on relationships and people, constant reprioritization of tasks as new ones land on my desk.

— **Kiran Mahon**

Exercise and get out into nature – there's a wonderful Japanese idea called "forest bathing" . Spending time outside in a quiet place lowers blood pressure and increases brain function.

Being organized - if you are less organized you are less likely to be able to deal effectively with emergent stressful issues while balancing the day-to-day. Schedule everything!

Deal with things in the moment – procrastination leads to growing task lists and added stress. Don't do it!

—Ross Maki

Stress is something I have paid attention to in my life for the last 10 years. It sweeps you away in the most subtle sort of ways. It prevents you from doing the things that truly keep you grounded and present with your day to day at work or in your personal life. Once that center is lost, it is easy to get swept away in the stress patterns and develop sabotaging behaviours that make it incredibly difficult to get back on track. Having lost my balance a few times along the way, here are some things that I do to stay present (as best I can anyway!)

Breath deep and breath often - When I am stressed my tendency is to hold my breath and my voice will come from my throat. Noticing is all that I need to do, and bring my breath back to my belly. For me that breaks the cycle of the stressful moment and brings me to self-care.

Recognizing less is more - When the work piles on and believe me we all know it can pile on, the first tendency may be to work harder, which I tended to do always. Unplugging and recalibrating is more effective for me now. I can navigate through the pile refreshed and renewed which allows me to put my best thought into the thing I am working on.

Bring myself back to nature - There is a grounding component to nature for me. Noticing the green in the trees, waves in the water, or the color of the sky even if it's raining has a tendency to snap me back. Taking a long walk in nature works wonders. Near my office there is a Golf Course and that has become a place where I go when I have those days, and they happen a lot! I retreat for a walk around the path. It is right off a main arterial road, but the large trees, bright green grass of the golf course and the crunch of the gravel under my feet bring me back to reality.

Spending time with my kids - Play is an underrated activity as an adult. My kids help me destress by helping me remember what play is. It is difficult at times, but I continue to work at it. I never try to say "No" when the kids ask me to do something. Whether it is playing with a box of Lego, or video game the kids like and I know nothing about, it allows me that moment to be a beginner. It reminds me that their relationships are what's important, not 300 emails in my inbox.

     —**Dave Lundberg,** www.smallpausecoaching.com

The main strategy that works for me is being mindful. Both practicing everyday mindfulness-in-the-moment, several times a day, and practicing daily meditation.

     —**Christina Nikiforuk**

High impact contact sports and listening to designated soothing songs.

     —**Taryn Scollard**

Leave your desk at lunch. Go for a quick walk to get some fresh air and clear your thinking.

—**Anne Nickerson**

When I was much younger I took a course through BCIT, the instructor was very inspirational and made an impact on me. I held on to some of the things he talked about and one was "walking and talking" to keep the blood pressure down......personally I think better when I am walking. Having "walking meetings" is something I started quite a while ago and has been a part of my management style for many years.

Beethoven, Darwin and Steve Jobs (to name only a few I'm sure) all believed in the power of walking. Being stuck in an office only makes me think of other "stuff" and I don't always focus on the person I'm talking to or the topic. Walking meetings refresh my mind, helps to keep me focused, allows me to be more creative and I feel it personalizes the connection between myself and the person I am walking with. Getting in a few extra steps during the day is a bonus health benefit (yes it helps for stress relief) that everyone can feel good about!

—**Howard Normann**

My strategies for handling workplace stress are: Bike commuting, going for a walk, talking to a colleague that has been through same experience, gardening, keeping my shoulders down and back and relaxing my breathing, talking to my spouse or a friend about the situation but telling the story as a comedy instead of as a stressful situation.

—**Dean McIntosh**